I0435296

The Natural Approach to Cosmetics and Personal Care That Won't Leave You Breathless!

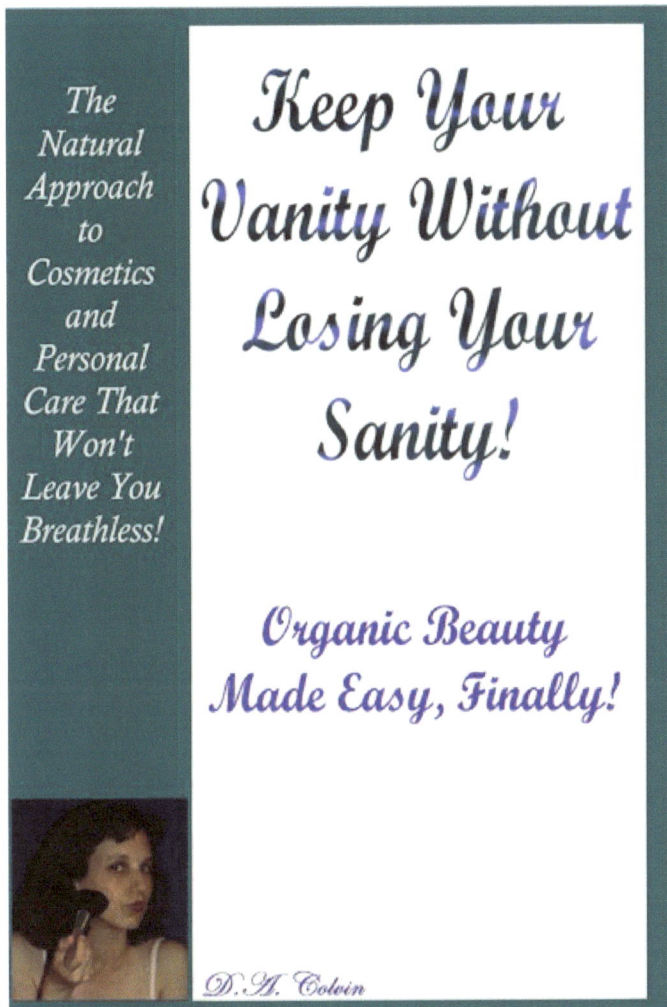

Keep Your Vanity Without Losing Your Sanity!

Organic Beauty Made Easy, Finally!

D.A. Colvin

Table of Contents

Please read this disclaimer:
The Health and Beauty tips presented in this book are not offered as prescriptions,
cures or otherwise. They are not to be taken as medical or dermatological advice. As with most advice,
you should not attempt to use any information without consulting your medical physician or dermatologist first.

Note: Some parts of this e-book may require being connected to the internet to access information.

Introduction

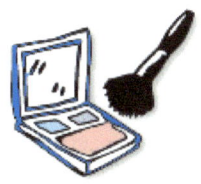

Chapter 1 – What Is Vanity?

Vanity is defined as extreme preoccupation with one's appearance. Vanity is the desire to look our very best – beautiful, sexy, handsome, and attractive. For many people, vanity is about having a "perfect, flawless" appearance. Vanity became an important part of the human condition when Hollywood and the film industry was in full swing during its heyday. Companies like Max Factor, Maybelline, Loreal, and Gucci began making products that every woman and man wanted in order to improve their appearance. These companies made products that helped men and women to feel beautiful and glamorous. During Hollywood's heyday, actors would spend hours in their dressing room choosing the right wardrobe for a particular scene. Actors would then have a makeup artist transform their plain faces into glamorous beautiful works of art.

Cosmetics and hair accessories have been a regular part of daily life for all walks of life in the Western World. Today, you rarely see an actor in the spotlight without makeup or a fancy hairstyle. Not only are these glamorous entertainers in the spotlight, but they often bombard you with commercial advertisements, both on television and in magazines, depicting themselves with glamorous makeup and fragrances. Advertisers create these obscene multi-million-dollar commercials in the hopes that the consumer will be hooked and not see through the veil of illusion. You have a world of vanity and glamour.

This is not to say that vanity is a bad thing. There's nothing wrong with looking beautiful and feeling glamorous and sexy. Who wants to walk around looking like something the cat dragged in or someone who looks as if he or she hasn't bathed in several days? We call it vanity because it is literally a preoccupation with one's appearance. The desire to have an attractive desirable appearance goes deeper than you think. It all comes down to two basic human elements – self-esteem and sex appeal. It doesn't matter whether you wear facial makeup, change the color of your hair or change your hairstyle.

The average person spends more than an hour a day improving his or her appearance. Couples throughout North America make it top priority to set aside a couple hours each day applying makeup, hair accessories, and the appropriate clothing before stepping out the door. Today, vanity is more complicated than ever because most men and women do far more than merely bathe and apply a little makeup. There's moisturizing cream, wrinkle cream, makeup for various skin tones, hair gel and mousse, hair spray, and hair tint and highlights. Essentially, men and women have made themselves glamour and fashion models for the outside world. They pay close attention to the commercials they see. They apply their makeup and style their hair just as the makeup artists and hairdressers do. They've made vanity a science of precision.

The reason behind this vanity is simple. There are two behavior elements that motivate all human behavior. People go to incredible lengths to avoid pain and gain pleasure. Men and women associate tremendous pain with looking ugly, dirty, and unappealing, so they go to unbelievable lengths to ensure a near-perfect appearance. Men and women spend over $100 in cosmetics and beauty supplies in the space of a month. There are times when $100 is the minimal. The more cosmetic improvements they want to make, the more money they need to spend.

When you think about it, vanity is an endless cycle of constant improvements because there's no end to the things people want to perfect. This is because it is human nature to care about what others think of us. Everyone has an opinion and we all tend to feel self-conscious about our appearance. So, it's only natural that we would go to such great lengths to ensure that we look our very best. This also stems from our childhood upbringing. As children, most of us grew up feeling very insecure. We wanted more than anything to gain the acceptance and approval of our peers. Regardless of whether we had a positive or negative self-image, it always mattered to us what others thought of us.

During the teenage years we feel the most vulnerable and impressionable. It would stand to reason that we would want to make sure that we made a weekly visit to the nearby pharmacy for all the latest colors, skin tones, and texture combinations. It didn't help that there were others in our age range that appeared to always have a perfect complexion and flaunted their good looks. These people always appeared to be very glamourous. For those of us who grew up very shy, awkward, and somewhat lonely, insecurity was our nature and we were always afraid that other people were looking down at us. This attitude carries over into the adult years. How many kids have watched their parents spend endless hours in the bathroom working on their makeup, hair, and clothing and grew up to perform the same rituals? It's a habit that continues with one generation after another. With more innovative products appearing on the market, there's always a desire to "keep up with the times" and have a fresh clean new look.

Vanity isn't merely limited to facial and hair appearance. Vanity encompasses everything that has to do with appearance. Fashion and facial structure play a very large part in vanity. In addition to cosmetics, fashion and facial restructure probably enjoy more than several billion dollars in sales each year. Between the cosmetic surgery men and women have done to their faces – nose jobs, facelifts, and Botox injection – and the liposuction and skin toning people have done, billions of dollars are spent each year on vanity. Today, you can't open the yellow pages in a phone book without finding thousands of plastic surgeons that perform these very surgeries.

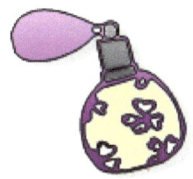

Chapter 2 - Perfume vs. Purefume

What happens when the products used for intimacy enhancement and self-improvement are toxic and repel the opposite sex? Imagine that the products you use to create a flawless model-like appearance do the exact opposite. Imagine these products creating health and skin problems that you actually tried to correct or prevent with these cosmetics. The multi-billion-dollar fragrance and cosmetics industries would have you believe that their products are safe, effective, and beneficial. The commercials that enter your television space every night depicting sexy models looking carefree and vibrant with their makeup would have you believe the same misconception. These commercials depict fragrances and cosmetics as a harmless beautiful addition to your beauty collection. What is the result of men and women using these cosmetics that seem so benevolent?

Fragrance and perfume products have been used for centuries for beauty, intimacy enhancement, and rejuvenation. However, the perfume that was in distribution before the advent of the Industrial Revolution was not the same perfume we use today. Yesterday's perfume is what we know today as purefume. Purefume is a term the Aveda Corporation coined to differentiate between toxic petro-chemical fragrance perfume and fragrances that are derived from pure plant essences – purefume. There is a world of difference between purefume and perfume. Purefume consists of pure organic essential oils that are derived from the life-blood of plants, shrubs, flowers, herbs, and bark. Pure essential oils are pure unadulterated plant essences that have been completely untouched and unscathed by man. Perfume, on the other hand, is one of the most toxic unhealthy poisons a person can use on his or her person.

Our natural bodily smells can be unpleasant and offensive, but toxic petro-chemical fragrance perfumes are a thousand times worse. The worst part about fragrance is that it is found in everything. It has made its way into every product we use for beauty, hygiene, household cleaning, and deodorizing. Whether you use shampoo, moisturizer, disinfectant, or face powder, fragrance will touch your life, but not in a good way.

The population has been turned into canaries in a coal mine. One of coal mining's earliest systems for warning of the presence of methane gas, the canary in the coal mine, though low-tech, was extremely effective and rather easy to read: if the bird died, miners had to get out of the shaft. Today, the citizens have become the canaries. We are the proverbial canaries in the coal mine, being used as guinea pigs by the cosmetics and fragrance industries. Every product ranging from shampoo and moisturizer to face powder and cologne is being tested on humans. What's worse is that this is being done without our knowledge or consent. If you were to combine all the chemicals used in cosmetics, plastic surgery, and Botox you could literally create an explosive bomb. These chemicals are toxic, carcinogenic, and contain petro-chemicals and irritants that create severe illnesses and respiratory problems.

According to the National Academy of Science as of 1999, more than 15% of the population suffers from fragrance and chemical sensitivity and cannot tolerate the exposure. That number steadily rises every year.

Environmental health awareness writer Andrea DesJardins states that the FDA does not regulate the fragrance industry. Andrea DesJardins also states that of the 5,000 different chemicals used in the fragrance manufacturing process, less than 20% have been tested for toxicity levels. Because there is no scrutiny, thousands of chemicals are used to manufacture fragrances. The result is a toxic witch's brew. Most people aren't aware of the toxic effect of these chemicals. Most people use these products blindly without even considering or being aware of the consequences.

A Harvard Study was conducted on the constituents and toxicity of fragrance products. According to this study, all fragrance products contain phthalates, a substance used in plastics. Phthalates are chemical irritants that cause adverse health problems, such as labored breathing, kidney, and liver malfunction. For more information, including a list of cosmetics that are unsafe and contain phthalates and those that are considered safe, please visit the website: www.nottoopretty.org. Studies have also shown that adulterated fragrance products contain pesticides, the same toxic petro-chemicals used to keep bugs away from crops. Once the genie is released from the bottle, the chemical demon comes out and torments us with its toxic poison. One of the detriments of using fragrance is that it's difficult to stop the usage. According to Anne Cheyne, contributing writer for the Camp Hill Medical Centre in Nova Scotia, Canada, the chemicals in the fragrance product desensitize the nerves and cells. What this means is that as a person uses the product, their nerves experience a dull-like sensation and become somewhat numb to the chemicals. When one is dowsed in fragrance, the scent weakens and the user's senses diminish. Those who don't wear any fragrance and are sensitive will immediately detect the scent. This would explain why fragrance users find it strange when a sensitive person is repelled by it. My husband and I endure this every time we have to go out and take care of errands. It's one of the reasons why I've had to restructure my life and work from home. The last time I had a job working under someone's employ I endured something I'll never forget.

I had a really cool job in the Pacific Design Center, known for some of the most famous renowned designers in the country. I started working for a designer and her assistant as their office assistant secretary and I was delighted and overjoyed. I had found a job that paid me decently with flexible hours and a boss who was fairly cool and easygoing. I was really excited. The first few days were pretty good. I performed the various tasks and did my job fairly well. I even started to develop a rapport with my boss. She was very kind and upbeat and I really enjoyed working for her.

One afternoon, I was sitting at my desk doing some work on the computer. The designer's assistant walked up to me while I was looking at the computer screen. Before I looked up at her, I started having trouble breathing and I smelled some horrible toxic stench that reminded me of a toxic hair salon. I held my chest and felt like I was going to die. I turned to look at her and find out what she wanted and then I took a close look at her hair. It was teased, perfectly styled, and appeared as if an entire can of hair spray had been used in it. Then, she opened her mouth and her cigarette smoke breath finished me. I couldn't breathe, talk, or move. I nearly collapsed to the floor, holding my chest for dear life. I couldn't decide whether to scream, cry, push and kick her away or bolt out of the office.

That's exactly what I did. I couldn't even breathe long enough to explain how I felt. I was so angry and horrified and scared because I really felt like I was going to die right then and there. As I bolted out, I could see that the assistant was watching me, wondering what was wrong. I wanted to tell the main designer what was wrong but I didn't think she would understand. I made a beeline for the bathroom and tried to regain my composure and my breath. I was horrified and could barely get my head together. Once I splashed my face and regained my composure, it was at that moment that I realized that I would never be able to have a normal job in a regular work environment again. I wanted to, but I couldn't because I knew that this was not an isolated problem. Everyone was into vanity and most people used all kinds of products to make sure their makeup and hair were perfect and stayed in place. I recount this moment every time I need to explain to someone what I go through and what it's like for someone like me with asthma and chemical sensitivities. It's true hell. It's a horrifying nightmare that only gets worse with the more toxic petro-chemical products being used. People who consistently use fragrance products don't know what it's like. They can't imagine how a person like me copes and suffers having to endure such toxic poison.

When watching commercials depicting sexy women covering their bodies with a beautifying product, your first thought is that your skin will feel just as young. You'll stop the wrinkles. Your new sensual feminine hair will glow with sexy highlights. Everlasting youthful beauty is the biggest motivation that keeps cosmetics sales on the rise. Now it's time to look at the listed ingredients. Usually, you'll see a long paragraph, indicating that this product you're using is loaded with ingredients. Chances are, those ingredients are toxic, especially the ones you cannot pronounce. There's a well-known expression that many health-oriented people live by when buying products. That expression is "if in doubt, do without". This simply means that if you don't understand the ingredient, you should avoid it. According to Anne Cheyne, one of the biggest problems is that many products claim to be "unscented" and "fragrance-free". Considering that this really isn't the case, this can confuse consumers. While the product may appear to be fragrance-free, the product is still scented and contains potentially toxic chemicals to the sensitive user.

One of the big culprits of this perfume problem is the advent of those discount "perfumery" stores that sell every type of fragrance, perfume, and crazy scent known to man. These aren't merely the regular scents that you would find in a department store or boutique. These are fragrances that were cheaply made with so many chemicals, alcohol, and horrible irritants, one could literally transform more than 100 new people into asthma sufferers in one moment. Fragrances today are made very cheap, fast, harsh, and overpowering. This would explain why several people who cross your path smell almost identical. My husband and I often find ourselves enduring this wherever we go. It seems that more and more people today are taking advantage of the "inexpensive cheap" fragrance impostors and are trying to smell like a glamour queen. What they're really doing is adding more toxicity to the air and they're making more people ill.

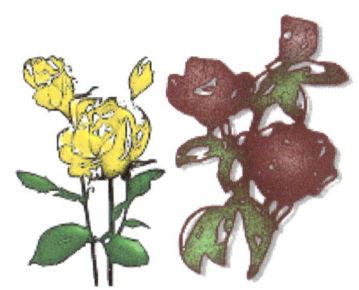

Chapter 3 - Pure Plant Essences

It's time for the million-dollar question. What's the solution to this toxic problem? Feeling appealing and having a high self-esteem are important. It's a natural instinct and should be nurtured in a non-toxic earth-friendly manner. Hygiene and cleanliness are basic needs. In truth, you don't need a dozen products for cleanliness. This is a fallacy. This is equally true for beauty. Try Aubrey Organics Honeysuckle Rose® Moisturizing Shampoo, a natural organic shampoo with extracts of Fennel, Hops, and Balm Mint. The solution to the intoxicating overpowering problem of toxic fragrances is so simple, many people don't see it. Some people see it, but they don't understand it and this is probably because the media does such a great job overwhelming us with their "amazing, wonderful, beautiful new products".

The solution is pure organic plant essences. Plants like cinnamon, lavender, patchouli, peppermint, rose, ylang ylang, and geranium are the sources for pure plant essences. Once in a while you'll cross paths with someone who smells so nice and natural and you can't identify their scent. It's like nothing you've ever smelled and yet it doesn't irritate your lungs or make your eyes sting. This is because the scent they're wearing is natural and pure. Pure essences have a completely different effect than those toxic petro-chemical derived fragrances. Plant essences lift you up, rejuvenate and do something far more important than fragrances do. They free your cells and keep you alert. They keep you from being desensitized. Once you stop using synthetic fragrances, you'll probably start to notice your senses becoming stronger and keener. This is because plant essences don't disguise or cover anything. They're real. They mix naturally with your own natural smell and essence for a balanced conjunction.

Another crazy incident happened to me that I'll never forget. This is one of those memorable events that left an indelible impression on me. I had to get my lungs checked and diagnosed for asthma by a lung specialist. I was very uncomfortable in his office, but I did what I could to maintain my composure in order to get diagnosed. The receptionist was covered in makeup with tinted hair and tons of perfume. The doctor was dowsed in cologne and between the two of them I thought I would die before he would have a chance to hear my lungs. While I was talking with him I pulled out a little bottle of an essential oil blend that I use to calm and relax my nerves. I had been suffering from lack of sleep and rattled nerves, so I wasn't feeling very well, but the oil blend helped me a great deal.

When it was time for us to leave the doctor's office, the doctor pointed out that the oil blend that I used smelled like perfume to him and bothered him. It was very strong and he couldn't tolerate it. My jaw dropped and I couldn't believe what I had just heard. As I was leaving I tried to plant a seed. I suggested that he try using Mia Rose Air Therapy products to keep the office fresh and the air clean, to which he arrogantly turned on his heel and ignored me without acknowledgment.

It was then that I realized that people who are accustomed to using toxic adulterated chemical products have very little tolerance for or desire to use natural essences. Their nervous system and cells have become so sensitized to the synthetic fragrances that the pure plant essences throw them off and create a so-called negative reaction. The other problem is that when these people are exposed to these pure oils they don't seem to feel any immediate effects. Over time with consistent use, the oils begin to affect their system, but it takes a great deal of consistent time. I realized that what was really going on was that they were experiencing a bit of a detoxifying effect.

There seems to be a great deal of controversy and conflict going on about synthetic petro-chemical fragrances and pure organic essential oils. Many people who suffer from multiple chemical sensitivity and asthma from exposure to harsh fragrances and chemicals would like to believe that all essential oils are bad and should never be used. This is because there are various essential oils being marketed that claim to be, but are not pure therapeutic-grade. In truth, these oils are adulterated, overly distilled, and many of them are diluted with water and/or alcohol. Some of them even have added chemicals, but the company would have you believe that it is a minute amount or something altogether different. The essence is literally being washed out and evaporated, so the healing properties never get the chance to work their magic.

Several years ago my husband and I met a peddler artist who was selling incense, essential oils, and semi-precious healing crystals. We got to know him and shared many things in common. I checked out his wares and took a whiff of his oils. I immediately felt ill and dizzy and I thought I would faint. I didn't understand what was wrong and I felt bad because this guy was really cool and kind and was trying to share his natural products with people. While incense isn't the greatest form of aromatherapy, it's far better than synthetic petro-chemical fragrances. I politely excused myself and later explained to my husband that the guy's oils were toxic and not pure. At first, he couldn't believe it and couldn't imagine that our friend would sell something toxic. Then, we realized that he didn't know they were toxic. I had thought of telling him, but street peddlers and artists tend to be a bit touchy and sensitive and I figured someone else would probably bring it to his attention.

The second time I was exposed to essential oils was in a famous metaphysical book store in Los Angeles that attracts people from all over the world. There was a display of various oil samples and I was intrigued. I was still learning and I wasn't familiar with most of them so I wanted to try them. The samples ranged from frankincense to sandalwood and they all smelled good. But the smells bothered me and agitated me and I was baffled. I didn't understand why essential oils that were touted as being pure and natural could bother me so much. I was disappointed because I was really enjoying learning about them and I had even considered buying a few.

A few years later, our dear friend introduced us to [Young Living Essential Oils](#) and I knew I was done searching. I tried a few of their oils and I was astounded. They smelled wonderful and created healing sensations in me unlike any other oil. I started to cry out of relief and I felt a strong emotional release. The samples of peppermint and tea tree (melaleuca) smelled so beautiful and powerful that this little whiff made me feel energized and rejuvenated for the remainder of the day. It was then that I knew that I would be a Young Living Essential Oils distributor and I wouldn't need to continue my search for better oils.

These were the best oils I had experienced and I was overjoyed. As I learned more about the company and all the wonderful oils, I realized the source of the controversy and conflict. I'm not about to criticize or speak poorly about oils from other companies, but the bottom line is simple. I have been fortunate enough to be exposed to a variety of oils from various companies, and it is clear which oils are pure therapeutic-grade and which ones are adulterated.

After thorough research, it was clear to me that these companies don't invest enough in the production of their oils. The organic plants are of the highest purest quality. They are all pure and unscathed. But the distillation process has omitted vital invaluable elements. The result is oils with a less than potent smell and healing property. I've heard some people say that the oils I use are expensive. My response is always that you get what you pay for. If you were to attempt to duplicate the stringent meticulous efforts and processes of Young Living Essential Oils, you would be grateful for the oils they provide.

Pure organic therapeutic-grade essential oils are priceless. These pure essential oils have helped me in many ways and have helped me to prevent major health problems. The controversy is so sad and makes pure essential oils like the ones my husband and I use look bad and toxic. If these oils were toxic and bad, we wouldn't use them. I'm the most sensitive person I know and I can detect an adulterated petro-chemical like a bloodhound. My senses can distinguish between something toxic and something pure.

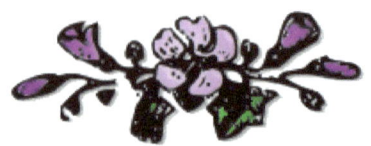

Chapter 4 - Earth-Friendly Plant Essence Cosmetics

It's important to vote with your wallet by shopping in a natural food store. When you buy mainstream chemically laden products from a mainstream store, you're doing much more than merely buying a product. Your hard-earned dollars are funding several ugly things that are hurting the environment, the social consciousness, and your future. When you buy a mainstream cosmetic beauty product, you're buying from a multi-national conglomerate that looks at you like a speck of dust. While the marketing companies occasionally provide discount coupons and promotional programs to save you money, it's all about marketing. The discounts have simply made the products more appealing to you. After all, how could you say no to something that saves you money? These companies exploit their workers and many of them have sweatshops. They have no interest in the environment or social justice. Their primary interest is profit margin.

At times, you may see advertising campaigns or special notes on a package that indicate that the product is partially recycled and that the company "cares about the environment". As horrific as this sounds, this is known as "green-washing". If you've ever seen the following commercial, then you'll understand what we mean. The scene opens up to the beautiful peaceful waves crashing on the beach with beautiful graceful sea gulls singing and gliding across the sky. You see turtles, marine mammals, and various other animal species gracing the sky and beaches, making it a perfect beautiful day. Then, you hear a male narrator discussing the importance of environmental responsibility and conscience. The last part of the environmental message you hear is "do people care about the environment and the creatures"? Then, a famous petroleum company logo insignia appears in the scene and you hear the words, "we do". Environmental and holistic groups refer to this as green-washing because that's exactly what it is. If you believe the message they're conveying, then you are not paying attention.

It is of no concern of theirs if the ingredients that are purchased for use in their products are of the lowest grade quality and kill laboratory animals. They don't care about recycling or environmental responsibility and they are in bed with the petroleum companies. See for yourself how heinous and ugly these companies truly are. Scratch one company and you'll find another that's even more powerful and greedy. Just do a search on the Internet for a manufacturer of a commonly used cosmetic product. You can see with your own eyes the ugliness that's behind it. A manufacturer of products that have no relation to the other makes many of these products you use. Why would you buy a lipstick made by a company that makes detergent or cookies? For more information, please see the list of sources in the "tools and resources" section at the end of this e-book. If this doesn't make sense to you and seems odd and ridiculous, then you're paying attention. If this doesn't bother you, then go right ahead and use this heinous product that probably destroyed more than 1,000 lives in the process. On the other hand, if this angers you, then keep reading and pay close attention. Your hard-earned dollars are going to give you a momentary feeling of beautiful self-confidence. The result will be endless aggravation and potential medical bills from the ill health you will suffer.

Beautiful model-like sex appeal doesn't have to be a toxic arduous task.

There are men and women throughout the world who enjoy sensual vibrant beauty without allowing one toxic substance to go anywhere near them. You too can enjoy this phenomenal beauty. It's much easier and far more cost-effective than one might imagine. If you want stylish lively hair, natural product companies like Aveda and Aubrey Organics have wonderful moisturizing products. These companies exude integrity and compassion for the public's health and that of the planet and animals as well. They don't conduct or condone the act of animal testing or environmental pollution. They refuse any studies or research that has involved animal testing and they don't accept low-grade ingredients that involve it either. Health and environmental responsibility are top priority to these companies. The healing herbal aromas are wonderful and a small amount is long-lasting. There's nothing like washing your hair and getting rid of the dirt and smelling like roses, cinnamon, or mint in the process.

If it's beautiful highlights you want, I would suggest consulting with an Aveda hairdresser. If dry skin plagues you, massage it with creamy moisturizing Aubrey Organics Rosa Mosqueta Hand and Body Lotion. Aveda colorful makeup is beautiful and aromatic. With so many beautiful colors, shades, tones, and combinations, you can have a lot of fun making your face, hair, and body look beautiful. You can create a look for nearly any mood and personality. You can create a silly playful look or a mysterious, provocative, sexy look. There really is no limit. The best part is that you're putting ingredients on your skin that are designed to improve your health and won't hurt you or the environment.

Imagine using an eye or lip pencil that smells like sandalwood, mint, or patchouli. It glides on so smooth and soft, you don't even know it's there. Imagine having these colors on your face without having to experience one ill effect or skin irritation from it. There is a pure plant essence-derived product for every single cosmetic, beauty, and hygienic need you have. If for some reason you do experience an adverse reaction, don't immediately panic or think the worst. If you've grown accustomed to using chemical mainstream products, this is bound to happen. Your skin and cells have grown accustomed to ingredients that are irritating and toxic and now you've switched to something pure and unadulterated. Sometimes a breakout or rash is simply a sign of a detoxifying cleansing effect. After a quick transition from using mainstream to natural products for so many years, my body and my skin began to react immediately. I was a little freaked out at first and I thought something might be wrong with the products I was using. Instead of jumping to conclusions, I calmed down and gave the products a chance to work their magic.

I had recently switched from the toxic mainstream products I was using to Aveda and Aubrey Organics. My skin began to tingle and felt alive and my hair felt as if it had been hydrated and oxygenated. All the chemicals had actually made it so my skin and hair could not breathe or get oxygen. I noticed a few irritations in various areas of my skin and I was concerned. But I intuitively knew that my skin was getting used to the new plant essences. After drinking plenty of water and applying some tea tree oil (melaleuca) to the irritations, they quickly disappeared and my skin felt more alive and free than ever. I was thrilled and overjoyed. I compared the toxic ingredient labels to the natural ones and there was no comparison. I was so grateful that there were companies like these that made such wonderful healing beneficial products.

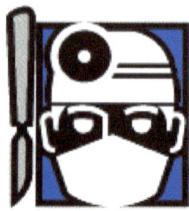

Chapter 5 – Cosmetic Surgery and the "Flawless" Appearance

We've entered an era where everyone wants the "perfect" flawless appearance. People will go to great lengths to shave at least 10 years off their age and transform their appearance into somebody they admire as a role model. They go to great lengths to create similar facial characteristics. One look at an awards ceremony on television is indicative of the billions of dollars celebrities spend in order to reverse the aging process and maintain a sexy young flawless appearance. This expensive obsession with vanity stems from a basic fear. Everybody is living with dread and fear of looking and feeling old and ugly. This reminds me of a profound song I heard, *Ugly Inside*, performed by *Mr. Jones and The Previous*. The lyrics are: "You're ugly inside, you're ugly inside, the beauty at the bottom is buried alive. You're so ugly inside, so ugly inside. That's a fact your makeup just can't hide."

This is the epitome of insecurity and vanity. Those who are so self-conscious and preoccupied with their appearance won't let anyone or anything get in their way of everlasting youthful beauty. They're all searching for and chasing the famed "fountain of youth" and they believe the so-called legend. What if all these people learned that the real "fountain of youth" is not merely a geyser spewing out water, which if drunk will create everlasting beauty? What if they learned that it is an actual process of mental and physical transformation?

My aunt, my dear uncle's widow, is one of these people who spent thousands and millions of dollars on her appearance. She spent the majority of her life living in Encino, California, one of the wealthiest, high society cities in the country, possibly the world. Encino is like Bel Air, Beverly Hills, Del Mar, or Carmel, also in California. It's a clean fancy city where the creme de le crème meet, dine, play, and work. You'll rarely see anyone looking plain, simple, dirty, or unkempt. You can call them snobs, conceited, or self-centered. These people live well and dress well. Some of the best-paid physicians, plastic surgeons, and lawyers live and work in Southern California.

My aunt was and is one of these high society people. When I was a young girl, she wore the classiest fashions and owned several boutiques. Every time I'd visit her at her boutique, there would be high society customers throughout the store and she was always busy consulting them on various styles. She spent more than half the time behind the counter ringing up bag after bag of clothes. She had several fashionable people working under her employ. I've always been curious about fashion and beauty, but I always questioned people for wearing such professional business clothes to work. I tried to understand why people spent so much money and time on makeup and their appearance. I would see people hustling and bustling about, looking for the "perfect" outfit and facial color combinations. I would wonder why these people couldn't just be content with keeping it simple and basic.

To this day, my aunt has spent thousands of dollars on fashion and makeup. She has probably had more than a dozen facelifts. It horrifies and astounds me that people will spend that much money and energy on their appearance when there are so many people throughout the world who are starving and can barely afford a meal for the day. I try not to judge or criticize, but people's priorities are truly backward. During crisis, what are these people going to do to feed themselves – eat their makeup and hair accessories and sleep in their fancy cars? Who knows? Maybe that's exactly what they'll do.

This is not to say that vanity altogether is wrong. It's not wrong and there's nothing wrong with wanting to look and feel good. Self-esteem is very important and we all need to feel loved, desired, and wanted. It's human nature. There's something very important to understand here. Some of the energy spent on vanity should be spent on looking deep within at our souls to the underlying reason behind our vanity. Why do we really feel the need to look so flawless and improve on something that may not need any improving? When we look deep within to our innermost being and see who we really are, our true inner feelings and desires, our true essence, we'll see more than meets the eye. We may even find there are deep emotional, even spiritual issues we're not dealing with and are using vanity to avoid dealing with them. I'm not a psychologist, but I know what it's like to focus so much attention on something unimportant, only to discover an underlying problem that's being neglected.

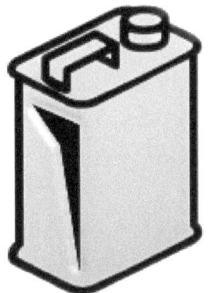

Chapter 6 – Gasoline On My Face!?

For years, I used baby oil on my skin to achieve softness. I would use a bar of soap that was touted as being a moisturizer and would make my skin feel like it was being gently touched and caressed. Then, I would put a few drops of baby oil on my face to add moisture. My mom turned me onto this ritual. My skin felt soft, smooth, and supple. But it didn't feel quite right. I couldn't put my finger on it, but my skin began to feel chewy and greasy and I detected a subtle fragrance. I didn't understand the feeling and I felt as if I were going crazy. I don't blame her because she didn't know any better, but I do wish I had learned then what I was fortunate enough to learn years later at an Aveda salon.

Contrary to popular belief, baby oil is not made from harmless minerals in the earth. It's fragrance and mineral oil, which is perfume and refined fossil fuels; in other words, dinosaur fossil bones. When I was told this, I nearly went into shock. I cried and I could hardly digest or believe what I was being told. I had performed this ritual twice a week for years and now I was learning that I had been putting refined petroleum on my face! Imagine my painful horror. Unsuspecting consumers perform the same moisturizing ritual everyday and use various other petroleum-derived products on their skin. I wonder how they would feel if they made the same horrible discovery as I did. I would imagine that these people would be outraged and horrified to know this. Who knows? Maybe, they would rise up and revolt against the multi-nationals that could care less about poisoning them, the animals, and the earth. But maybe not, considering that most people rarely question anything they're fed and taught.

Another product that's used everyday is what is commonly known as the brand, Vaseline (TM®). This is a petroleum product people use to moisturize and lubricate. Now, think about this for a moment. What is Petroleum Jelly? Well, if it doesn't seem obvious to you, then perhaps an explanation is in order. If you take a close look at the word, it might occur to you that it's a jelly made from Petroleum or sometimes referred to in ingredients as Petrolatum. To reiterate, this product is derived from the same petroleum that gasoline is made from, in other words, the stuff you pump into your gas tank. There are several ingredients found in cosmetic and hygiene products that are derived from petroleum. Paraffin, petrolatum, mineral oil, polyethylene glycol (PEG), and propylene glycol are common toxic petroleum-derived ingredients found in today's cosmetics. There is nothing beautiful, healthy, sexy, clean, or natural about using petroleum on your skin or in your hair. If you think that there is, then you need to read further and learn the truth. If you find this disgusting, then perhaps you would like to learn more about this and look into natural alternatives that won't make you potentially flammable.

Let's examine the basics of petroleum. Petroleum is a dark, oily, flammable liquid found in the earth's crust, consisting mainly of a mixture of various hydrocarbons; coal oil. Yes, that's correct. Petroleum is the smelly, dark, disgusting stuff that's refined and processed into gasoline, the clear smelly stuff you pump into your gas tank. You may ask why companies would put such disgusting toxic ingredients in products used to beautify, clean, and improve your appearance. Petroleum is a multi-billion-dollar industry. You'll find petroleum by-products in nearly every product man uses for cleaning, lubricating, painting, polishing furniture, and beauty. Why would an ingredient that's used for lubrication be put in cosmetics? Good question, I'm glad you asked! Petroleum is a cheap commodity that's in high demand. You can see evidence of this with the gas price hike at the gas station. This has been a serious controversy since the holistic organics movement began in the early 70's. Companies got the crazy idea of using petroleum by-products as an inexpensive lubricant in cosmetics instead of using something non-toxic and biodegradable.

Now, you may ask, what can be used in place of petroleum? What's beautiful is that there is zero need for this toxic, greasy, smelly stuff. There are many plant products to choose from to replace petroleum. Jojoba is a plant found in Mexico and parts of the Southwestern United States. Jojoba is a wonderful plant that is used as a lubricant and is found in various medicines. Jojoba is found in many natural plant-derived cosmetics. It is a wonderful oily lubricant and has a pleasant smell. Sesame, grape seed, olive, and soy oil are other seed oils that are used for lubrication and are very effective as massage oils. Some people like to mix them for a nice pleasant smelling potent healing massage. Another wonderful product that's great for moisture is rose water.

Many years ago, my husband and I attended a natural product show in Anaheim, California and were introduced to some wonderful natural products. I was still in transition from using chemical products and wanted to make sure I was using the best products for my health. That's when I was introduced to Rose Water and some wonderful natural products that are simple, effective, and economical. I was given a sample of rose water to splash on my face.

At first, I was a little skeptical and I wasn't sure if it would work. The next day, I washed my face with an Aveda(TM®) facial cleanser and I put a few drops of the rose water on my fingers and rubbed it into my skin. Wow! I was amazed, floored, and once again cried tears of joy. It smelled great. It felt great and I was in love. I never knew that rose water could be so moisturizing and clean. I then cried because I was wishing that I had known about this when I was using baby oil on my skin. Thank goodness for my common sense and waking up to the realization that I could use natural products for all my needs.

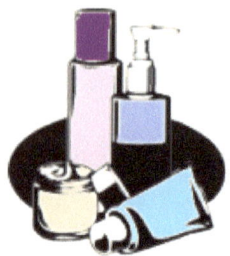

<u>Chapter 7 – FD&C's, PEG, and Propylene Glycol</u>

If you had difficulty with pronouncing the name of this chapter, you're not alone. While label reading is a science, it's not always a pleasant one. No one said reading labels was going to be easy or pleasurable. The one thing it will do for you is it will save your life and will show you what you are putting in and on your body. Think about it this way. Let's say that someone gave you something to drink or put on your face without informing you of the contents. Then, you used it and it was revealed to you that it was poisonous. Would that bother you? If you are a normal thinking feeling human being, then of course it will bother you. Only a masochist or suicidal person is willingly going to consume something that they know will make them ill.

Knowledge is power. There is nothing more powerful than knowing exactly what you're being exposed to and the effect it will have on you. When I first learned that mineral oil was essentially produced from the same stuff gasoline is and was toxic to my health, I was horrified and devastated. I also wasn't stupid. There was no way I was going to let anything like that touch me again and I was committed to being a strict label reader. Reading labels is very empowering. It makes you feel strong, powerful and aware and gives you the strength and courage to take charge of your health. Those who either aren't accustomed to reading labels or refuse to do so will suffer the consequences of their willful ignorance. Even if you're in a hurry, taking an extra minute or two to read a label is crucial. If those extra minutes feel abhorrent to you, then you probably shouldn't be buying the product.

Every product that you see on the shelf in the store has the potential to benefit and improve your health or make you very ill. You have the power to decide what goes in and on your body. You have the power to decide whether you will feel good and alive or sick and miserable. All the power lies in your hands and your wallet. There are three common ingredients found in most cosmetic and beauty products. These three ingredients are extremely toxic and are largely responsible for many of the health problems in this world. FD&C's, also known as Food, Drugs, and Cosmetics, are named for the various synthetic food dyes you find in food and cosmetics. You also find them in medication, hence the chemical code name. When you read a product label and see ingredients like "red 40", "blue #8", "blue lake #4", or "FD&C blue lake #40", you're looking at suspected highly toxic petro-chemical food dyes. These dyes are also derived from coal tar and they may cause cancer, mutate the blood cells and can make you feel miserable.

When you are shopping for food, take a look at the baked desserts and ice cream. If the food seems unusually vibrant and colorful and doesn't look natural, you're correct. Those colors are synthetic petro-chemicals and will possibly make you very sick if ingested. These things are better off as wax candles than as food. When the cosmetic beauty product you're considering buying looks very colorful and vibrant, chances are this product is laden with toxic food dyes. Polyethylene glycol (PEG) and propylene glycol are two other toxic petro-chemicals that are carcinogenic and found in nearly every cosmetic beauty product. They are even found in some foodstuffs. PEG is a chemical compound of chemical plastics. Propylene glycol is essentially the same thing. Both are used in anti-freeze and lubricants and are highly toxic. You may ask the question again. Why are these ingredients used in food and cosmetics? Like the other toxic ingredients that are mentioned in this e-book, these are cheap commodities used and distributed by the petroleum industry. It's simple and easy for these industries to mass-produce them in consumable products.

You probably won't smell or taste these petro-chemicals, but you will feel their effects in your body. They don't feel good and they don't benefit your body in any way. They are potentially very harmful. You can ask questions and analyze this until you're blue in the face. You can also express your anger and move on and start buying sensible and beneficial products. This is what my husband and I did when we learned the truth. We felt angry, upset, disappointed, betrayed, and disgusted. We continued to peruse the information before us and shared our knowledge with those who were receptive to it. We used our disdain and passion to impart our knowledge to others. We continue to do our best to help prevent more people from being intoxicated and polluted.

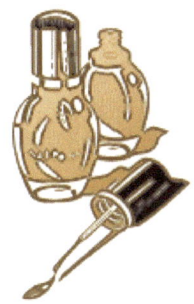

Chapter 8 – Non-Toxic Beautiful Nails

Nail care is another part of vanity that contributes to ill health and environmental degradation. Healthy beautiful fingernails and toenails are as important as a clean beautiful complexion and clean healthy hair. People spend as much time, energy, and money on their nails as they do for the rest of their body. Salons that provide manicures and pedicures enjoy a great deal of business because men and women need to have flawless nails. Add nail color polish, chemical treatment, and fake acrylic nail tips to the basic maintenance and you have a very expensive beauty regimen. It's important that your nails are as clean, groomed, and attractive as the rest of your body, but there is such a thing as overkill.

In some of the wealthier parts of the country, I've seen women and teenage girls of all ages (as young as 13) flaunting their vanity. Wherever I went with my friends as a young girl, whether it was the movies, shopping malls, or restaurants, I would see women and teenage girls looking like they had just stepped out of a beauty salon. Their hair would be professionally styled without a hair out of place. Their makeup and skin were perfect and flawless. Their clothes were clean, upscale, and wrinkle-free, and their fingernails always appeared perfect.

Women wouldn't just have their fingernails cared for – they'd give equal attention to their toenails. Women and teenage girls would have this done just for the fun of it when going about their daily activities. They weren't going to a special party or dinner engagement. They just did it because it made them feel beautiful. Again, everyone wants to feel beautiful. It's human nature. But when everyone starts wanting to emulate fashion models and celebrities who have assistants cater to their every whim, things get out of hand.

Having healthy pretty nails is just as simple and easy as having healthy clean hair and skin. It just depends on your standards and what you consider to be healthy and attractive. Ten years ago, I tried the vanity beauty thing for a bit and I enjoyed it a little. But I was never the type of girl who enjoyed putting a great deal of attention on her appearance. It just wasn't me. I've always been very down-to-earth, grounded, and simple. Sure, I would not leave the house looking like a ragamuffin, but I didn't feel the need to resemble a fashion beauty queen. I'd spend maybe 20 minutes or so brushing my hair. I might wet it a little to get rid of frizzies or flyaway hair. Then, I'd splash my face, put on some clean clothes and a little pretty jewelry and I was ready to step out the door.

On my 21st birthday, my friends thought it would be cool if I got a professional manicure with fake nail tips. As a receptionist secretary, I typed all day on a computer keyboard, answered phones, and handled various office machines. So, I wasn't sure it was a good idea. I decided to do it because all the other girls looked so good with their pretty fake nails. I was going through a phase where I still felt unsure of myself as a woman. I hardly knew any women or girls of any age who had plain ordinary looking nails, except for my mother and grandmother. I went with my friend to a nail salon she frequented and prepared for the big moment. I still felt unsettled and even a little silly. The idea of having my nails done was ridiculous and stupid to me, but I figured this once it would be okay.

The first thing that offended me was the plethora of toxic chemicals I had to breathe. I started wheezing and felt very dizzy and my head hurt. That didn't stop me. The sweet girl concentrated all her attention on my small fingers and transformed my plain simple little nails into shiny long masterpieces. I still felt silly, but I was blown away and couldn't help but notice how beautiful they looked. I had half-inch nail tips extending from my little fingers and my hands actually looked more adult. They felt and looked beautiful. When I was done, I wondered how long they would last. I soon discovered that in order to have these beautiful nails, I would need to have them maintained and filled every two weeks. For those who don't know what a fill is, it's the process of adding more acrylic powder and chemical gunk where the nail has started to grow. In other words, they fill it in with more powdered acrylic junk. There are many nail styles you can choose from and they're all very pretty – French tips, squared, rounded, decorated, and pretty color shades. You can have the same thing done to your toenails.

As wonderful and feminine as this all sounds, when you step back and take an objective look at it, it's absurd. The process of cleaning the hands and pushing back the cuticle, followed by polishing the nail is an arduous task. Add to that the process of applying that gross toxic acrylic junk with the plastic nail and you have tremendous physical pain. When I had it done, the novelty lasted for about two days and then I regretted it. I'm a very active person and I do many things with my hands throughout the day. One of those things is writing. I spend a lot of time during the day writing. Can't you tell? I'm the author of this e-book and I typed it all. When I had nail tips, fastening a button or moving something with my fingers became an arduous task. I had to ask my husband to help me with things because I was afraid my nails would break. Sure enough, that's exactly what happened.

One after another broke. I cried and I was upset. At first, I was going to spend the money to have it done again, but I decided it wasn't worth it. As pretty as they were, I needed my fingers and I wasn't about to stop being an active productive person. I enjoy being pampered, but I've grown accustomed to doing things on my own. I grew up learning how to feed myself and brush my hair and I don't need someone to do that for me. I'm not criticizing those who do the very thing I'm against, but I think it's silly to get all dolled up, especially when you're the only one who can enjoy it.

The process of caring for the nails is harmful to your health and the environment and it's big business. Walk into any pharmacy, market, and discount store and you'll see the money people spend on nail care. There are kits that enable you to do it on your own without the aid of a professional. It's just more toxic smelly glue to smell and irritate your lungs. What would the world be like if these salons disappeared and everyone was forced to be natural without fake shiny nails and glamorous Farrah Fawcett or Jennifer Aniston hair? Have you ever noticed the natural radiant beauty of a nature-inspired artist when dressed in colorful flowing garb? She or he may not have beautiful nails, but your attention is drawn to the eyes and their beauty is timeless. He or she smiles and you can see into the soul. The naturally clean hair flows easily and dances with the gentle breezes. The skin has a radiant glow and the teeth exude good health and hygiene. This is real natural earthy beauty. Unscathed, untouched, and unpolluted by the 21st century.

The natural non-toxic remedy for healthy strong beautiful nails is simple. If you want your nails to be healthy and strong, you must care for them from the inside. For starters, discontinue the toxic chemical products you're using because they're only going to make your problems worse. If you're concerned about splitting, chipping, or peeling, then you need more calcium, which is found in leafy greens, nuts, seeds, grains, and nut butters. If your cuticles feel or look unhealthy, perhaps it's the chemicals you've been using. Rather than focusing on keeping your nails looking shiny, pretty, and fancy like everyone else's nails, try a more wholesome down-to-earth approach. Your nails may not shine or look like they belong to a young beauty queen, but they'll be healthy and strong and that's what matters!

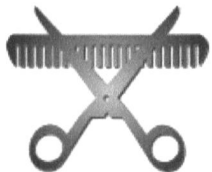

Chapter 9 – Beauty Salons – A Toxic Soup

Beauty salons play a significant role in vanity and the pursuit of the "fountain of youth". You can find a beauty salon in every city and town across the country and throughout the Western World. For every beauty and cosmetic need, there's a salon ready to serve that need. Some salons cater to every aspect of beauty, including shampoo and haircut, makeup, color, tint, and style, while some cater to more specific beauty needs. Walk into any of these salons and you'll see men and women being transformed into model-like beauty. You'll find more people seated in the waiting room waiting for their transformation. There is no question that beauty is big business in the Western World. You can get a professional shampoo and haircut, style, color and tint, massage, manicure and pedicure. You can even have your bodily hair waxed and removed. Men and women spend a tremendous amount of time and money having their appearance transformed and altered.

It is nice to be pampered once in a while. It feels great and is relaxing and good for the soul. It feels wonderful to have someone massaging your scalp, washing your hair, and beautifying and massaging your skin. It's heavenly and feels wonderful! There's nothing like it. When done in a holistic, non-toxic, earth-friendly manner, being professionally pampered does wonders to lift the spirits and create an overall sense of well being and good health. When done in an environment that's uncomfortable, toxic, and hazardous to your health, it can be a nightmare that will leave you walking out in tears, gasping for your next breath.

Considering the poor indoor air quality, beauty salons are suspected to be large contributors to asthma and other respiratory conditions. It's amazing that with the overpowering ammonia and other toxic smelly chemically-laden beauty products being used, anyone can walk in and out without fainting or being rushed to the emergency room. It's not so much that salon proprietors don't care that they're endangering the public's health. Some beauticians aren't aware of the health hazard and are focused on maintaining their business and happy clientele. They don't have the time to investigate healthier means of cosmetic beauty. Perhaps they do have the time, but skepticism prevents them from making a change. In addition to the products the cosmetologists use on their clients, they use toxic unhealthy products on their own hair and skin. It's a vicious cycle. But it doesn't have to be that way.

Walk into any Aveda Concept Salon and you'll experience something altogether different. Aveda Corporation was founded by Horst Rechelbacher, an Austrian environmental health pioneer whose mission and goal was to improve the quality of life on earth for the people, the animals, and the planet. To learn the whole story about Aveda, you can visit their web site at: www.aveda.com. Aveda's products utilize pure plant essences and are known as plant kinetics. The company has stringent strict standards as to the type of people who distribute and use their products and the type of atmosphere and environment a salon creates. You will rarely walk into an Aveda Concept Salon and feel depressed, agitated, dizzy, or aggravated. Each salon owner hires only the best men and women to provide professional health and beauty services. My husband and I have visited several concept salons and they are all very nice, clean, peaceful, and conducive to healing relaxation. In addition to the services they provide, it's also a wonderful opportunity to receive an education on personal health and environmental awareness. I am not here to sell Aveda and I don't work with them. However, if all, but Aveda salons disappeared and the only option was Aveda salons, the world would be much better.

One of the aspects I like best about Aveda concept salons is that the estheticians are not permitted to use cosmetic products other than Aveda. Most of them are so enamored with Aveda, they have no interest in anything else. These wonderful estheticians take personal and planetary health very seriously and are in complete support of holistic and organic beauty. Each time I've gotten a haircut from an Aveda stylist, I always hear the same thing. They detest petro-chemical synthetic fragrances and perfumes as much as I do. They use and enjoy only Aveda products.

When I was younger before the days I began learning about holistic natural living, I would go to one of the little franchise haircut places. These are the places where you can get a haircut for less than $20 without an appointment. You walk in and give the receptionist your name and the type of service you want. He or she writes down the service with the price on a receipt next to the others in line ahead of you. Then, you sit down and wait for your name to be called. Because my hair grew like a weed I had to get it trimmed every couple weeks so it wouldn't grow long like Pocahontas. I always got a kick out of going to these places and enjoyed the novelty.

Then, I began learning about the toxicity of petro-chemical synthetic products and I no longer had the desire to get my hair cut at any of these places. I started to notice the noxious smells emanating from the salon products, as well as the stylists and customers. I no longer enjoyed going there and I then realized that you really do get what you pay for. Granted, there are many Aveda salons that charge in upwards of $60 and much more for a shampoo and haircut, but there are some that charge as little as $20 or $30 and I've been to those salons. Not everybody is financially wealthy and can afford an expensive haircut. For those who can, there's no reason to spend your money on professional beauty services that are toxic and harmful to your health and the planet.

Remember that you don't just vote with your wallet at the market. You also vote with your wallet at the salon. When you spend your money on a haircut and style performed by someone wearing and using toxic products that are harmful to your health and the environment, you are saying that these things don't matter to you. Conscious spending is very important. It doesn't matter if you're buying shoes, vegetables, or a facial. When you spend your money on a professional non-toxic haircut at an Aveda Concept Salon, you're doing a wonderful conscious thing. Your money is going to a salon that truly cares about the health of the people and the planet. That money is used to keep the salon healthy, healing, and harmonious. Doesn't it feel better to spend your money in a place that has a conscience and cares about the environment? There is no contest.

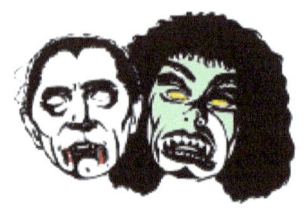

Chapter 10 – Halloween

Next to Christmas and Thanksgiving, Halloween is one of the most celebrated honored holidays of the year. It never ceases to amaze me how many people get into the spirit of the holiday and enjoy the festivities. 2,000 years ago, Halloween was a very sacred holiday celebrated by the Celtic people in the ancient British Isles. It was a holiday celebrated by Druids, Witches and Wiccan Covens, Fairies, Elves, and various other Celtic tribes. On All Hallows' Eve, as it was called back then, the Druids would go from door to door holding an empty basket asking for fruit and whatever treats the residents would give them. Later in the evening, everyone would gather together in a festival, dancing, singing, playing, and enjoying the foods they were given.

Many centuries later, Halloween is still a celebrated holiday, but today things have drastically changed. People still enjoy wearing costumes, pretending to be their alter ego. They also enjoy going door to door saying, "trick or treat" and asking for sweet treats, but the tradition has vastly changed. Halloween is probably one of the most expensive holidays. As soon as the summer begins to fade, stores begin stocking up for Halloween and the Christmas Holiday Season. Throughout the store, you'll see the regular merchandise combined with racks upon racks of new Halloween paraphernalia.

One of the biggest traditions of Halloween is the wild and elaborate costumes people design. Many people go with the traditional Angels, Ghosts, Devils, and Superheroes, while others opt for outlandish costumes, portraying celebrities in Hollywood. The costumes are usually cute, colorful, and beautiful and the makeup is a process all to its own. Dressing up and playing make believe, pretending to be someone or something else for a day is fun and exciting. It is a beautiful way to express the inner child. The problem is that the makeup and hair goo that is used to complement the costumes is usually toxic, smelly, and very harmful to the health. It's fun to dress up and wear wild and zany colorful makeup and create funny wild hairdos that get attention. But when these products contain toxic petro-chemicals, the fun disappears.

I remember attending Halloween parties with friends and I always had a great time dressing up and checking out everyone's getup. We always had such a great time trying to guess what someone was supposed to be and admiring the elaborate costume designs. Unfortunately, there was also a down side. Each person had bright or dark colorful thick makeup on and colorful hairspray with funky silver and gold streams sticking out of their hair. As soon as I would get close to someone, I would have trouble breathing, would start coughing, and I'd make a mad dash for the bathroom. At first, I thought I was crazy and I couldn't understand what was wrong until years later.

When my husband and I began learning about holistic natural living, we began to question and analyze all the holidays. We were invited to a couple parties, but we started turning down invitations. I was no longer interested in wearing funky or sexy costumes with wacky colorful makeup because I couldn't find anything fun that was non-toxic. All those crazy facial makeup applicators and the silver and gold aerosol junk you put in the hair are permeated with toxic petro-chemicals. That shiny silver and gold stuff that you use to draw lines and decorations around your eyes and on your cheeks is filled with petroleum, potentially toxic food dyes, and horrible fragrance. It's cheap and massively distributed to all cheap dollar stores and can make people very ill.

If you want to have fun and get dressed up in some wild funky colorful costumes and makeup, opt for something that is safe enough to eat. Aubrey Organics and Aveda make some beautiful makeup, including some playful, funky, wild colors. There's no reason that you can't have fun in a non-toxic earth-friendly manner. The cheap inexpensive little makeup applicators you find in the bargain stores are better off ignored. A really good way to enjoy Halloween and the Holiday Season is to make your own non-toxic earth-friendly makeup and check out some books with some good non-toxic tips. Check out the resources section at the end of this book for some great holiday makeup ideas.

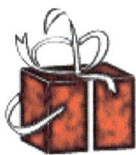

Chapter 11 – Christmas and the Joy of Giving

Christmas is one of the most beautiful celebrated holidays of the year. It's the most sacred, honored, cherished holiday and it tends to bring out the best and even the worst in people. Christmas is about giving, sharing, and being with those you love and cherish. Christmas brings out the festive spirit in people, inspiring them to bring out the Christmas trees, decorations, beautiful music, and lights. There's also the desire to get dressed up and look your best and give special beautiful gifts that make your loved ones smile. I remember countless family gatherings at the dinner table. I would look around the room at all the people I had grown to love, feeling so grateful for the love and everything they'd given me. Then, I would notice how dressed up everyone was and they were all covered in colorful makeup. My aunt in particular always appeared as if she had just stepped out of a boutique and beauty salon. Except for home videos showing her as a pretty young wife and mother in a natural manner without makeup, I don't remember ever seeing her plain, natural, and simple. She was always a glamour queen and that's the image people associated with her.

When it came time to exchange gifts, there was always such anticipated childlike excitement in the air and everyone anxiously waited to see what they had received. I was always so happy and excited that I would tear open my present without enjoying the pretty wrapping and packaging. I was usually given some neat pretty things that would improve my wardrobe or some playful things to wear in my hair. Other times, I was given things to use in a bath. Sometimes, I was given colorful makeup. I didn't mind it. In fact, I thought it was cool and I loved the pretty colors inside the compact case. But the smell always bothered me.

During a visit with my grandmother several years ago, she offered to give me a couple bottles of bubble bath and liquid soap someone had given her. Since the bottles were pretty and pink and she knew I had always enjoyed taking a bubble bath, she thought I would enjoy it. I wanted to tell her that I couldn't handle fragrance products and the chemicals inside would make me ill. Instead, I took a quick look at the bottle and cringed at the long list of chemicals. I simply said that it was a nice thought, but I had plenty of beauty and bath products. She looked at me kind of funny and probably thought I was a bit odd, but she smiled and nodded. She wasn't about to insist upon my using something that would make me uncomfortable. I thanked her for the nice gesture and suggested that she give it to someone who would enjoy it. She tossed it in the garbage, which upset me, but I let it go.

Giving is a wonderful thing and it can be something magical to enjoy for many years to come. Kind thoughtfulness is the key to giving. Whether it's a hand-crafted knitted purse or a special personalized decorated bottle with your friend's name on it, the joy of giving is something to be cherished and appreciated. Those who know me and are close to me know that the best things to give me are those things that are natural, organic, and earth-friendly. My friends know it's best to give me a recycled handmade card that they scented with a pure organic essential oil. What's equally important about giving is the way you spend your money. When you give to someone you care about, let them see that you care where your money is spent. Let them see that your only interest is in contributing to the solution, not the problem. Show them that you are only interested in supporting those companies that are socially and environmentally responsible. Giving is a magical beautiful thing and it should be done with the purest loving heart.

Chapter 12 - The Hundredth Monkey

On an island far away, there lived a tribe of monkeys that lived apart from the outside world. They lived their daily lives in the same manner every day and enjoyed their peace and solitude. Every day, they ate yams in the same manner - sniffing the aroma and eating them, without washing them. Every monkey continued this basic ritual all day every day throughout the islands. One day, one of the monkeys on one of the islands decided to do things different and change the eating ritual. Instead of not washing and sniffing it, he decided to just wash it. This was a strange new phenomenon and the other monkeys observed this odd new behavior. At first, the other monkeys just watched, baffled and amused. Then, one of the observing monkeys decided to try the same thing and a few more became intrigued until almost the entire island was following suit. Before long, every monkey on every island in this tribe was performing this ritual and had changed the traditional manner in which the yams were eaten. This became a famous well-known phenomenon throughout the world and was recounted by Ken Keyes, who authored *The Hundredth Monkey*.

The principle behind this story is the concept of word of mouth. It's been said that the best form of advertising, marketing, and promotion for business is word of mouth through those people you know. This is true and very effective. It's also true for vital knowledge and wisdom that can positively affect change in the world. Everything in this world becomes a fad, trend, and popular habit due to rumors and steadfast word of mouth. While Madison Avenue is the top advertising giant in the world, word of mouth is just as effective, beneficial, and powerful. This is one of the reasons that some companies opt for the avenue of network marketing and direct sales because they know that "the hundredth monkey" principle is very effective and powerful.

The hundredth monkey principle applies to everything in life. It is the best way to get a vital message across to other people in the most expedient way possible. Because of the billion-dollar conglomerates that target impressionable citizens with their manipulative advertising and marketing, citizens have to make a strong positive influence on those close to them. These vital messages have to be carried from one person to another in order to reach a critical mass. Unfortunately, there are many people in this world who are asleep and naive to the wolves in sheep's clothing. It's up to the aware ones to wake them up and educate them. It's terribly unjust when someone possesses wonderful knowledge about something important that can positively impact the world and doesn't share it with others who need it.

The only way we are going to be empowered and strong is to send a strong message to those heartless multi-nationals that we don't want their poison any more. We are ready to think for ourselves! How else do you think you can get through to a corporation that is greedy and faceless and doesn't even know you're alive? Silence will bring several dozen more discount perfumeries on every block peddling poison to the unsuspecting ones you love. The power is in your hands and the choice is yours. You possess the power within you to make a difference and make a positive change!

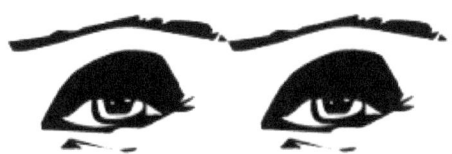

After Thoughts

No one has the right to dictate the actions or choices of another person. People have the blessing of free will to make the choices that make them happy. However, courtesy and consideration are very important. The Golden Rule that we learned in elementary school applies here. Doing unto others as you would have done to you is not an outdated ridiculous principle. It's a principle that people throughout the world continue to respect. We all have our own personal space or bubble around us. Anything that we do or use on our person is our personal choice and affects only us, providing that it stays within that space. Many people try to live by that, but wind up using fragrance products that are overpowering. Sometimes they use too much of it, which results in the vapors affecting the people around them.

For people like myself who have developed a painful sensitivity to fragrance products, the best thing to do is maintain an open receptive mind and be willing to learn something new. If you want to smell good and pretty, check out some pure therapeutic-grade organic essential oils. Treat yourself to some scents that complement your personality. If you want to maintain a beautiful or sexy look, check out those products that will effectively do the job in an earth-friendly non-toxic manner. It's easier than you think and it can be a win/win situation. You can enjoy your timeless youthful beauty and those around you can enjoy the non-toxic earthy scent that you exude.

When you want to smell appealing and feel rejuvenated, organic essential oils like geranium and sandalwood are wonderful. There's an essential oil for every mood, season, and occasion. [Young Living Essential Oils](#) (see the resources section in this book) make the best quality pure therapeutic-grade essential oils on the market. When searching for cosmetics, look for familiar ingredients like geranium, lavender, sandalwood, and rose essential oils without the added chemicals. With wonderful healing natural products like the ones recommended in this e-book, there is no need to look any further for cosmetic and beauty needs.

We've entered an era where a discount perfume central is at nearly every city block and it's almost impossible to not be exposed to it. Every store you walk into has aisles and racks of cosmetics, beauty supplies, and hygiene products beckoning you to take them home and fill your air with their scents. If you're fairly new to the toxic vs. non-toxic worlds, it can be overwhelming and a bit confusing. Providing you can understand what you're reading, it can actually be an enjoyable learning experience. There's no reason for anyone to suffer and there's no reason for ignorance. Between the Internet, alternative news media, printed published media, and books, there is truly a bounty of information available at your fingertips. All you have to do is maintain an open receptive mind and be willing to hear the message.

For every beauty need, there's an effective organic plant-derived product that will enliven your skin and make you feel wonderful. Your local natural food store has an array of products to try. The right one will appeal to you. All you need is an openness to learn. The sky's the limit and your health is worth it!

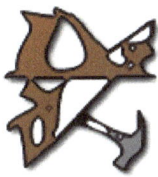

Tools and Resources

I want to thank you for taking the time to read this e-book I've compiled. This is one of the most important works I've ever completed. I really put my heart and soul into every word. I know how challenging and even painful it can be to learn something that's completely "out of this world". It can sometimes feel like learning a new language, especially when it goes against and challenges all your childhood and lifetime beliefs. To this day, I can remember how I felt and reacted the first day that I was introduced to natural organic living. At first, it challenged everything I'd been taught, but as soon as my inner intuitiveness and common sense kicked in, the challenge had turned into a hunger for knowledge that couldn't be quelled. I've always been the type of person that once I learn something that makes sense and challenges the very core of what was ingrained in me, I stop and listen.

The concepts, tips, and recommendations in this book are merely suggestions and don't have to be followed to the "T". Everything in this e-book is factual, accurate, and can be validated on the Internet and in books and printed media. My primary purpose for writing this book was to share my personal experiences and my perspective and give you the wherewithal to fully understand the way the world of cosmetics and fragrance operates. Being lied to, deceived, manipulated, and tricked is one of the worst cruelest things that can be done to a person. Unfortunately, this is the very thing that Madison Avenue spends billions of dollars each year doing. Commercials do a good job of this and this is why people, such as my husband and myself, either turn off the TV or mock and laugh at the stupid commercials that try to get inside our heads. I hope this e-book touches your life in a beautiful way and helps you discover what's real. I hope it helps you on your path of learning and self-discovery and empowers you to make wise intelligent decisions and choices! From my heart and soul, D.A.!

The following is a list of books, magazines, and web sites to help you along the way:

Sources:

Environmental Health Association of Nova Scotia
Andrea DesJardins
FDA
Harvard Phthalates Study
Mineral Oil
Petroleum Jelly
Propylene Glycol
Polyethylene Glycol (PEG)
FD&C

EPA Study

Web Sites:

http://www.notperfume.com   Not Perfume – raises awareness about the toxicity of perfume and fragrance products.

http://bodyearthself.blogspot.com Green Goddess - Enjoy a Healthy Chemical-Free Life! Articles, prose, and recommended books about environmental awareness and natural living.

Young Living Essential Oils   makes 100% pure therapeutic-grade organic essential oils. There's a therapeutic-grade essential oil for every mood from A to Z. **When ordering, please use member #252264, thank you.**

Aubrey Organics   Aubrey Organics makes a complete line of cosmetics derived from 100% pure plant essences from all over the world.

Aveda Corporation   Aveda Corporation makes a complete line of cosmetics derived from 100% pure plant essences from all over the world.

http://www.safecosmetics.org Campaign For Safe Cosmetics.

http://www.miarose.com Mia Rose makes wonderful Air Therapy products made from 100% pure citrus essential oils, Vanilla Beans, Spruce and Fir and nothing else!

http://www.fpinva.org Betty Bridges, R.N., provides a bounty of vital information about the FDA, cosmetics, and toxic fragrances. This web site is an incredible eye opener! Be sure to take some time to study the information on it!

Author's bio

D.A. Colvin is a social and environmental issues writer and is a very active environmental
advocate and animal rescue advocate. She and her husband live on the East Coast of the USA
and share a home with two adorable, wonderful, sweet cats, their babies. D.A. is a natural living
expert and offers advice to those who desire to live healthier greener lives.
Contact D.A. at via her website at: http://bodyearthself.blogspot.com

other Helpful Books: recommended.

Drop-Dead Gorgeous: Protecting Yourself from the Hidden Dangers of Cosmetics

The Truth About Beauty: Transform Your Looks And Your Life From The Inside Out

Natural Organic Hair and Skin Care, Aubrey Hampton, President and Founder of Aubrey Organics. Aubrey grew up on a beautiful farm in a small town where various types of plants and herbs surrounded him. His mother taught him to have an appreciation for the natural and herbal world around him, thus was the beginning of Aubrey Organics. This book is available at Aubrey Organics.

Eating For Beauty "Will open your eyes to the hidden treasures of a healthy diet and open your body to a fulfilling and vital existence"

Back To Eden Jethro Kloss, grandfather and founder of the natural living holistic movement. This book contains everything you need to know about non-toxic, healthy, simple living. It's a bible for natural living. Don't leave home without it!

Reclaiming Our Health: Exploding the Medical Myth and Embracing the Sources of True Healing, John Robbins, author of the best selling *Diet for a New America*. *Reclaiming Our Health* tells it like it is and reveals the truth about the medical industry that others are too gun-shy to reveal, but is aching to be told!

Other Helpful Resources:

5 Secret Tibetan Exercises To Tone Your Muscles And Gain Energy!

Please Send in Your Fragrance Stories, both Good and Bad. It might just find its way into our next book!

CREDITS
Images Courtesy of Designed to a T
Song Lyrics, *Ugly Inside*, *Mr. Jones and The Previous*

www.ingramcontent.com/pod-product-compliance
Lightning Source LLC
Chambersburg PA
CBHW040313010626
45792CB00022B/290